Lynda AOUDIA

Molecular signatures of breast cancer

Lynda AOUDIA

Molecular signatures of breast cancer

Mammography-ultrasound correlation

Imprint

Any brand names and product names mentioned in this book are subject to trademark, brand or patent protection and are trademarks or registered trademarks of their respective holders. The use of brand names, product names, common names, trade names, product descriptions etc. even without a particular marking in this work is in no way to be construed to mean that such names may be regarded as unrestricted in respect of trademark and brand protection legislation and could thus be used by anyone.

Cover image: www.ingimage.com

This book is a translation from the original published under ISBN 978-620-6-71281-7.

Publisher:
Sciencia Scripts
is a trademark of
Dodo Books Indian Ocean Ltd. and OmniScriptum S.R.L publishing group

120 High Road, East Finchley, London, N2 9ED, United Kingdom
Str. Armeneasca 28/1, office 1, Chisinau MD-2012, Republic of Moldova, Europe
Printed at: see last page
ISBN: 978-620-7-68464-9

MOLECULAR SIGNATURES OF BREAST CANCER: MAMMO-ULTRASOUND CORRELATION

LYNDA AOUDIA

FOREWORD

The molecular classification of breast cancers defines cancer subgroups with distinct molecular profiles and different prognoses and responses to treatment.

Studies have looked at the imaging appearance of each tumour subtype: radiologists need to be familiar with these to adapt the management of an aggressive subtype.

In the light of current knowledge, the following are observed significantly more frequently: a spiculated mass with a peripheral echogenic halo in luminal subtype A; architectural distortion in luminal subtype B; an irregular mass with an indistinct border containing microcalcifications, with an abrupt interface on ultrasound in the HER2 subtype; a lobulated mass with an indistinct or microlobulated border, very hypoechoic, with an abrupt interface, sometimes pseudobenign, in the triple-negative subtype.

The aim of this book is to provide an understanding of the molecular classification of breast cancer and the therapeutic strategies adapted to each tumour profile, as well as illustrating the mammographic and ultrasound aspects of each tumour subtype.

Professor Lynda AOUDIA

TABLE OF CONTENTS

INTRODUCTION

Breast cancer is a highly heterogeneous disease with different molecular profiles, depending on the presence or absence of oestrogen receptors (ER) and progesterone receptors (PR), and whether or not the HER2 gene (Human Epidermal Growth Factor Type 2 Receptor) is amplified. The cancers therefore have different prognoses and response to treatment [1, 2].

Imaging plays an important role in the diagnosis, staging, treatment and follow-up of breast cancer patients, and can also help predict the molecular subtypes of breast cancer in order to guide management.

Expression profiles have made it possible to define tumours with different prognoses, opening the way to therapeutic strategies tailored to the tumour profile, and even to prediction of therapeutic response.The more aggressive subtypes of breast cancer are more difficult to diagnose - some imaging features mimic benign lesions and may therefore be overlooked on standard imaging.Numerous studies have looked at the imaging aspect of each tumour subtype, which the radiologist needs to know in order to adapt management.

1. ANATOMICAL REMINDER

Mammary glandular tissue is made up of around twenty lobes. Each lobe is made up of 20 to 40 lobules, each with a galactophore duct, into which the secondary ducts drain, each leading to a ducto-lobular terminal unit (DLTU), consisting of a terminal duct, collecting several acini (fig. 1). The alveolus or acinus takes the form of a small, rounded sac. Microscopically, it is made up of two types of cells, the milk-secreting epithelial cells and the myoepithelial cells responsible for contraction, which rest on a basement membrane in direct contact with the blood capillaries (fig. 1).

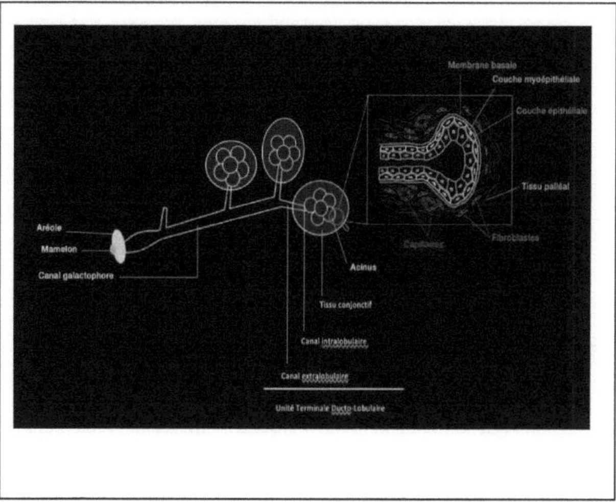

Fig. 1: Schematic representation of the components of mammary gland tissue.

2. HISTOLOGICAL BACKGROUND

Nearly 95% of malignant tumours are carcinomas, meaning that they develop from the epithelial cells of the mammary ducts and lobules. Sarcomas and lymphomas are rare, and intramammary metastases exceptional [3].

2.1. Stage of breast cancer

There are several stages in the development of breast cancer, carcinoma in situ and invasive carcinoma (fig. 2).

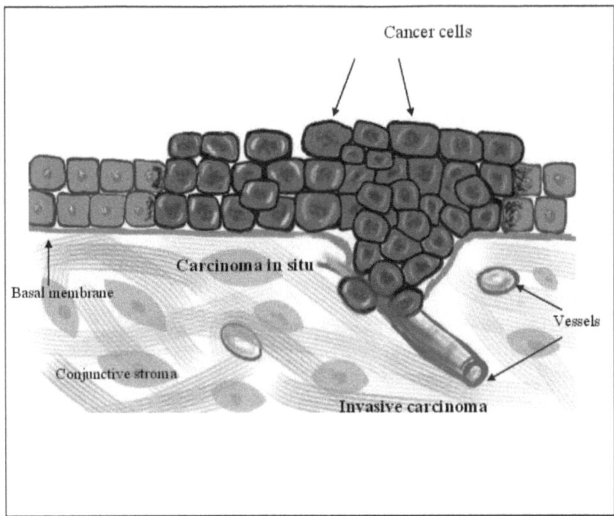

Fig. 2: In situ and invasive breast carcinoma.

2.1.1. Carcinoma in situ

In situ cancer is defined as a proliferation of malignant tumour cells limited to the interior of normal epithelial structures and which have not crossed the basement membrane, without metastatic potential.

2.1.2. Invasive carcinoma

Invasive carcinoma is a cell proliferation which, having crossed the basement membrane, infiltrates the surrounding breast tissue. Among the many histological entities recognised by the WHO, two major groups stand out: the non-specific form, formerly known as infiltrating ductal carcinoma, which accounts for around two-thirds of all infiltrating cancers, and the other so-called specific forms [3].

2.2. Histopronostic grade

Three parameters are assessed and scored from 1 to 3 to determine the histological grade of the tumour:

1. The architecture of the infiltrating cancer may or may not reproduce the architecture of a normal breast,
2. the appearance of the nuclei, the degree of anisonucleosis or the extent of nuclear inequalities; this is estimated by reporting the percentage of regular or irregular and monstrous nuclei (0 to 25%; 25 to 50%; more than 50%),
3. the number of mitoses in 10 microscopic fields at magnification 400.

The sum of the scores gives a total of between 3 and 9, defining three grades: 3 to 5 corresponds to grade I with a favourable prognosis, 6 to 7 to grade II with a moderate prognosis and 8 to 9 to grade III with a poorer prognosis. Ellis and Eston modified the Scarff-Bloom-Richardson (SBR) score to improve reproducibility (table 1) [4].

Différenciation architecturale	Proportion de structures tubulo-glandulaires dans la tumeur	
	Score 1	Bien différencié (> 75 % de la tumeur)
	Score 2	Moyennement différencié (10 à 75 %)
	Score 3	Peu différencié (< 10 % de la tumeur)
Pléomorphisme nucléaire	Atypies nucléaires	
	Score 1	Noyaux réguliers entre eux et de taille inférieure à 2 fois la taille de noyaux de cellules normales
	Score 2	Critères intermédiaires
	Score 3	Noyaux irréguliers avec anisocaryose ou de taille supérieure à 3 fois celle de noyaux normaux, avec nucléoles proéminents
Mitoses	Comptage des mitoses sur 10 champs au fort grossissement, rapporté au diamètre du champ (abaque de Elston et Ellis, ici pour 0,57 mm de diamètre)	
	Score 1	0 à 9 mitoses
	Score 2	10 à 18 mitoses
	Score 3	> 18 mitoses
Grade histopronostique	Score total obtenu en additionnant les 3 items	
I	3 à 5	Pronostic favorable
II	6-7	Pronostic intermédiaire
III	8-9	Pronostic défavorable

Table 1. Scarff Bloom Richardson histopronostic grade modified by Elston and Ellis [4].

2.3. Molecular classification

Breast cancer is a highly heterogeneous disease with different molecular profiles, depending on the presence or absence of oestrogen receptors (ER) and progesterone receptors (PR), and whether or not the HER2 gene (Human Epidermal Growth Factor Type 2 Receptor) is amplified, with different prognoses and responses to treatment [5-7]. This classification was first described by Prat and Pérou in 2000 [8]. It was established on the basis of genetic data on breast tumours (fig. 3) (table 2).

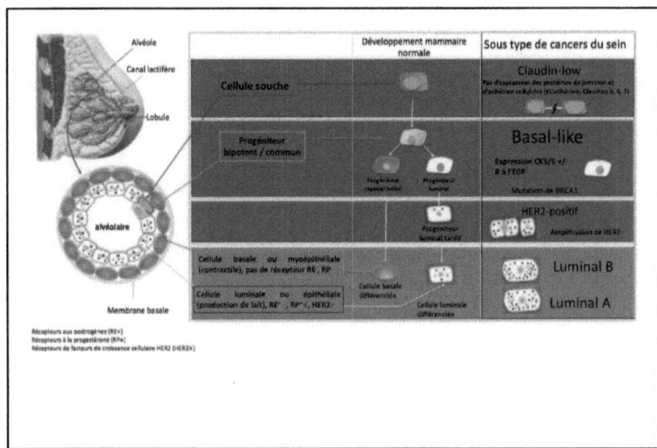

Fig. 3: Hypothesis of tumour development according to the molecular subtypes of breast cancer according to Prat [8].

Sous type moléculaire	Immunohisto-chimie	Incidence	Pronostic	Thérapie
Luminal A	RE +, RP +, HER2- Ki 67 bas < 20 %	50 - 60 %	Bon	
Luminal B	RE +, HER2- Ki 67 élevé ≥ 20 % / RP	10-20%	Intermédiaire	Chimiothérapie / Anti HER2 / Hormonothérapie
Luminal B-Like	RE +, HER2+, Quelque soit RP et Ki 67		Intermédiaire	
HER 2 +	RE-, RP -, HER2+	15 - 20 %	Péjoratif	
Triple-Négatif	RE-, RP -, HER2-	10 - 20 %	Péjoratif	

Table 2. According to St. Gallen International Expert Consensus 2013 [9].

2.3.1. Luminal type A

It accounts for 50-60% of breast cancers. It is characterised by high expression of oestrogen receptor (ER) and progesterone receptor (PR) genes, high expression of ER-regulated genes (GATA-3, FOX A1, etc.), low expression of proliferation-related genes and absence of HER2 overexpression. P53 is mutated in 13% of cases. This molecular type expresses proteins from cells located towards the lumen of the ducts, hence the name "luminal". Immunohistochemically, this type corresponds to infiltrating carcinomas expressing ER and RP with a low Ki67 proliferation index of less than 14% (fig. 4).

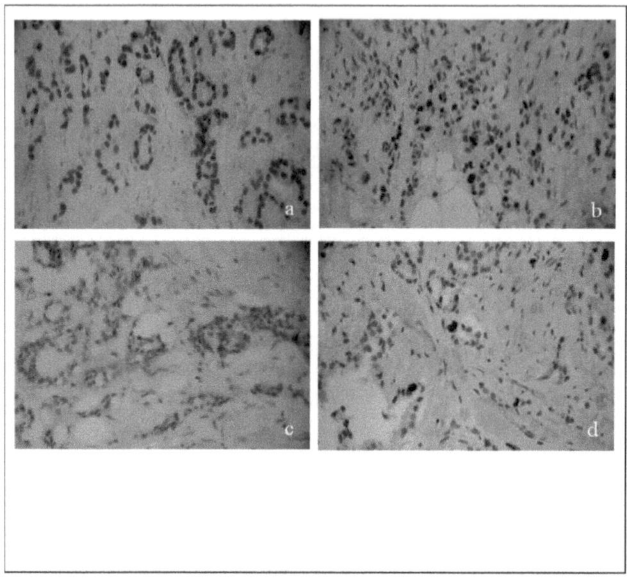

Fig. 4. Luminal A. (a) ER immunohistochemistry, ER positive. (b) Immuno-Histochemistry RP,RP positive. (c) Immunohistochemistry HER2, No HER2 overexpression. (d) Ki 67 immunohistochemistry, Ki67= 6%.

2.3.2. Luminal type B

It accounts for around 20% of breast cancers. Compared with luminal group A, it has lower expression of ER genes, lower expression of ER-regulated genes (GATA-3, FOX A1, etc.), and high expression of proliferation-related genes. P53 is mutated in 66% of cases. In terms of phenotype, this type corresponds to infiltrating carcinoma expressing ER and RP, with or without HER2 overexpression and more or less a high Ki67 proliferation index of over 14% (fig. 5).

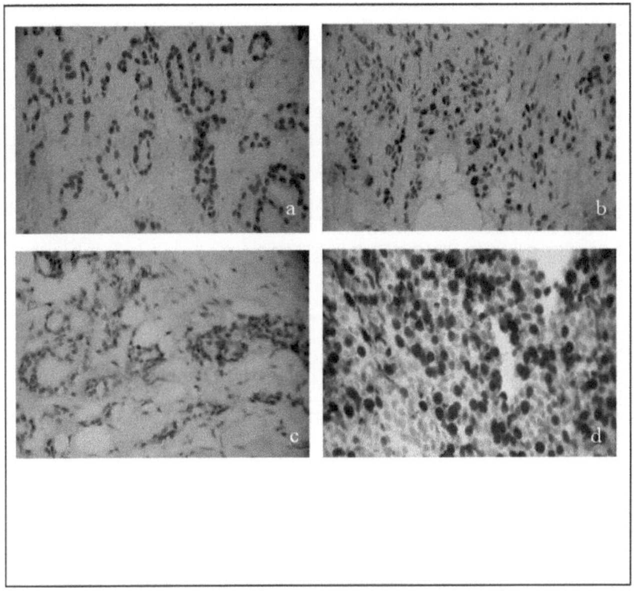

Fig. 5. Luminal B. (a) ER immunohistochemistry, ER positive. (b) Immuno-
(b) RP histochemistry, RP positive. (c) HER2 immunohistochemistry, No HER2
overexpression.(d) Ki 67 immunohistochemistry, Ki67= 60%.

2.3.3. HER2 type

HER2 cancer accounts for 10% of breast cancers. It is characterised by overexpression and amplification of the HER2 gene on chromosome 17q12, overexpression of the Her2 oncoprotein and lack of expression of ER-related genes. P53 is mutated in 71% of cases. Immunohistochemically, this type corresponds to infiltrating carcinoma not expressing ER, with HER2 Score 3+ or 2+ in FISH, whatever the Ki67 (fig. 6).

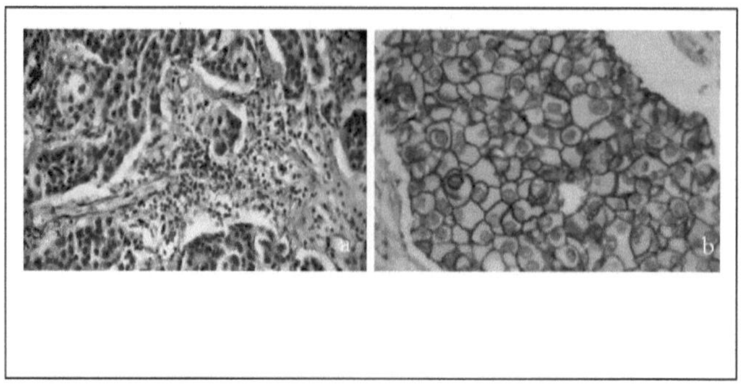

Fig. 6 HER status. (a) Microscopy, CCI. (b) HER2
immunohistochemistry.HER2 overexpression.

2.3.4. Triple negative type

It accounts for 7-16% of all cancers, and 70% of tumours occur in BRCA1-mutant women [10, 161]. It is characterised by a complete absence of expression of the ER and progesterone gene and HER2, hence the name "triple negativity", associated with strong expression of the genes for high molecular weight cytokeratins type 5/6 or 14 and EGFR (epithelial growth factor receptor). In terms of phenotype, this type corresponds to infiltrating carcinoma expressing neither hormone receptors nor HER2.

Mammography Technique

Mammography is the benchmark radiological examination for screening for breast cancer, which is the leading cause of death in women. Mammographic images must be optimised in terms of spatial resolution, contrast and noise. Several technical criteria must be taken into account, in particular, the contrast must be high in order to visualise microcalcifications properly. The radiation spectrum must be broad in order to adapt to the varying densities of the breasts and the minimum radiation dose, particularly in young patients.

3. POSITIONING

Positioning the breast is a fundamental stage in mammography, and the technique must be beyond reproach. The aim is to radiograph the entire mammary gland, including the deep planes. Positioning is the key to obtaining images of optimum quality, which are essential for interpretation and meet a number of quality criteria [12].

3.1. Fundamental impacts

3.1.1. Front or cranio-caudal view

The X-ray beam approaches the breast craniocaudally (fig. 7).

Difficulty of frontal incidence

In the absence of visualization of the deep mammary planes, it is important to engage as much posterior mammary tissue as possible.

Good incidence criteria (fig. 8)

The breast is in the centre of the image. The gland is well spread out.

The nipple is at its zenith [13]. No folds or overlaps.

The pectoralis muscle is visible in almost 30% of cases, and its presence on the image allows optimum depth gain [12].

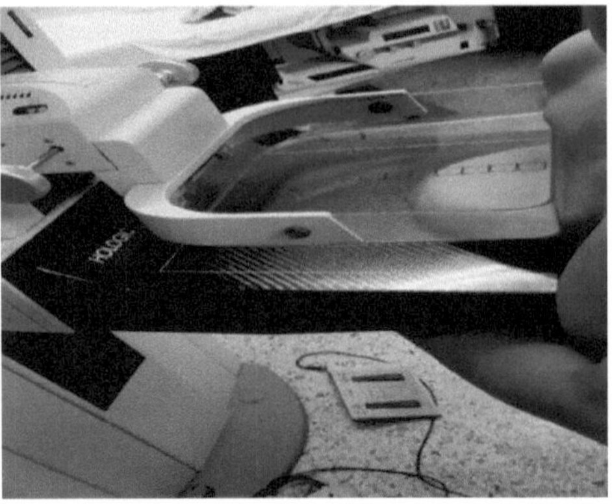

Fig. 7: Frontal or craniocaudal incision.

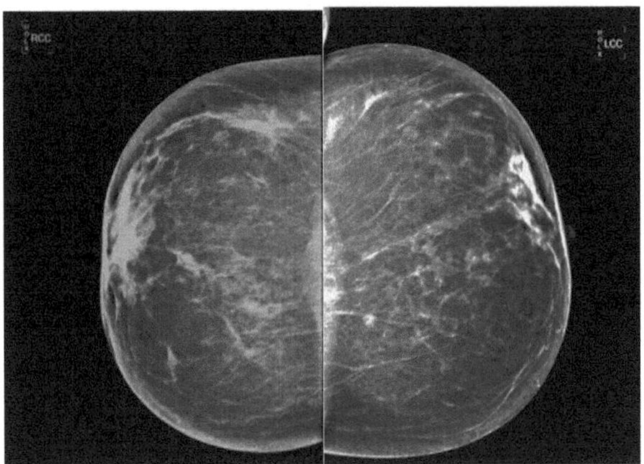

Fig. 8 Quality criteria for the frontal view. Mammographic images. (a) Right side. (b) Left side. Pectoral muscle (1), nipple at zenith (2).

3.1.2. 45° external oblique incidence°

This angle allows the breast to be studied in its long axis and a maximum amount of breast tissue to be analysed [14]. The stand is tilted at a strict 45° angle° , to ensure reproducible views (fig. 9).

Difficulty of oblique incidence

Compress the pectoral muscle, breast and submammary fold evenly.

Good incidence criteria (fig. 10)

The pectoral muscle is visible up to halfway up the image [15]. The nipple is at the zenith, opposite the tip of the pectoral muscle [14]. Presence of the skin fold of the abdominal wall [13].

The long axis of the breast tends towards the horizontal. Presence of the "open" submammary fold, perfectly clear of the abdominal wall [16].

No creases or overlapping.

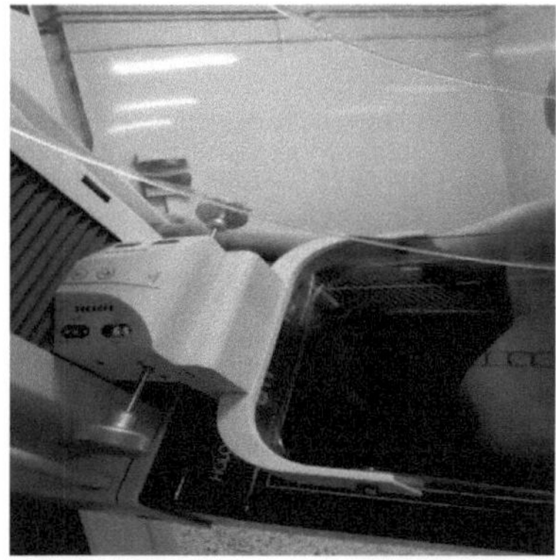

Fig. 9: External oblique incision.

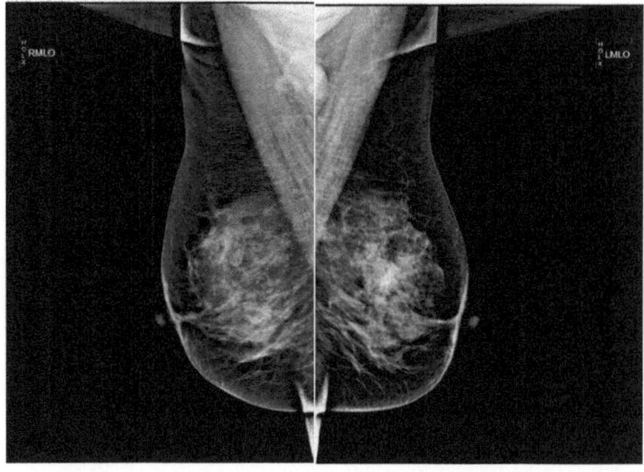

Fig. 10 Quality criteria for external oblique incidence. Mammographic images (a) Right oblique (b) Left oblique. Pectoral muscle (1), skin fold of the abdominal wall (2), open sub mammary fold (3),nipple at the zenith (4).

3.2. Additional impacts

They are always carried out in addition to the fundamental impacts.

3.2.1. Profile incidence

It is useful for determining the precise location of a lesion. It can also be used to show whether microcalcifications are located in a horizontal position.

3.2.2. Centred localized image

It can be used to analyse the contours of a nodule or a stellar image, or to eliminate a constructed image (fig. 11).

3.2.3. Enlarged centred image

Microcalcifications visible on standard images can be enlarged for detailed analysis (number, appearance, organisation, etc.) (fig. 12).

3.3. Other impacts

Axillary extension, Cleopatra incidence, staggered frontal incidence, tangential view, Eklund manoeuvre [17-20].

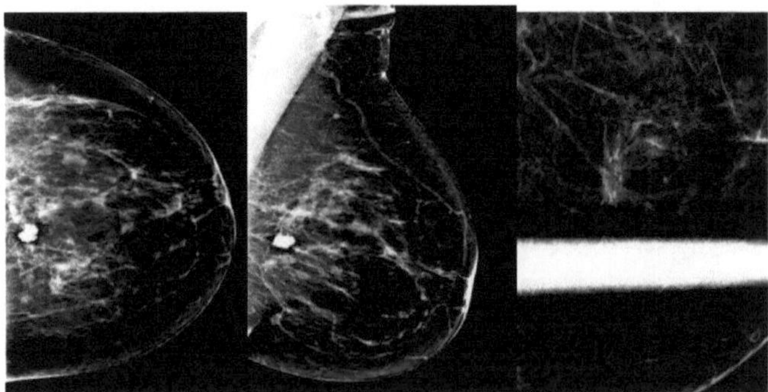

Fig. 11. centred localized view. (a) Front view. Mass with indistinct contours (arrow). (b) External oblique view. Mass in the sub mammary fold with poorly defined contours (arrow). (c). Centred view located on the mass. Spiculated mass, BIRADS 5 (arrow).

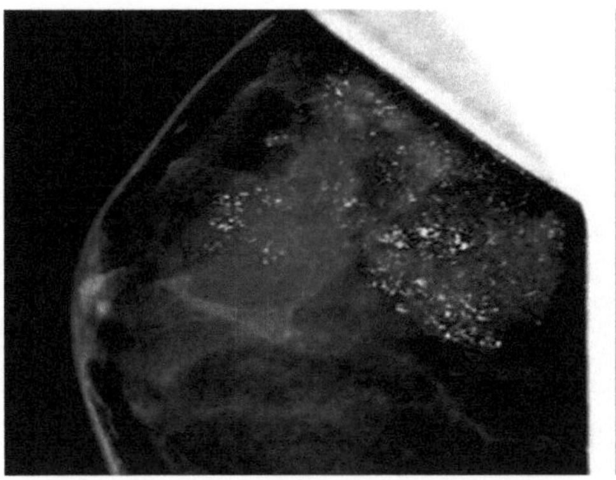

Fig. 12. Enlarged centred view. Magnification of a focus of micro-calcifications.

Ultrasound

Ultrasound is an accessible, non-irradiating and inexpensive imaging technique. It may be indicated as a complement to mammography, to improve lesion detection, particularly in dense breasts, and to characterise lesions, in particular to differentiate between solid and cystic lesions, and to take samples [21].

Breast ultrasound is performed with a high-frequency probe, usually between 9 and 15 MHz, which provides good contrast and spatial resolution [22]. There are several ultrasound modes.

4. MODE B

This is the first technique used when performing breast ultrasound. Ultrasound waves are emitted and collected by the probe, at the same frequency, in a single direction. They are combined to create a 2D image of the breast on a greyscale [23]. This technique allows structures to be differentiated on the basis of the acoustic and mechanical properties of the tissue. This B-mode has a number of weaknesses, including inconsistent optimal resolution and artefacts that can degrade image quality [24] (fig. 13).

5. HARMONIC MODE

It is linked to the non-linear behaviour of breast tissue in relation to ultrasound. As the ultrasound wave propagates through the breast tissue, it undergoes progressive distortion of the shape of the ultrasound pulse, creating harmonic frequencies which are multiples of the emission frequency [25-27]. Once the initial signal has been filtered, the harmonic signal is used to reconstruct the image. This technique improves the contrast of ultrasound images, particularly for cysts with "thick contents" or complicated cysts, which show internal echoes in B mode, whereas in harmonic mode they appear anechoic [28] (fig. 13).

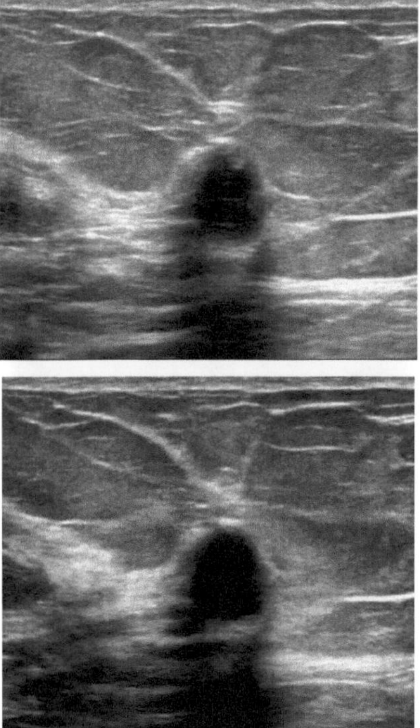

Fig. 13: Harmonic mode (a) B-mode ultrasound, hypoechoic mass, (b) Harmonic mode ultrasound. Cystic anechogenic mass with thickened wall. Histology. Histology: remodelled cyst.

6. COMPOSITE MODE (COMPOUND)

There are two types of composite, frequency composite (several different ultrasound emission frequencies are used to reconstruct the final image), and spatial composite (several ultrasound emission angles are used and combined into a single composite image). This technique makes it possible to limit artefacts, improve analysis of lesion contours, better define the internal echostructure of masses and detect small lesions [29] (fig. 14). It also allows better detection of intra-lesional calcifications [30]. On the other hand, posterior ultrasound changes are attenuated [31].

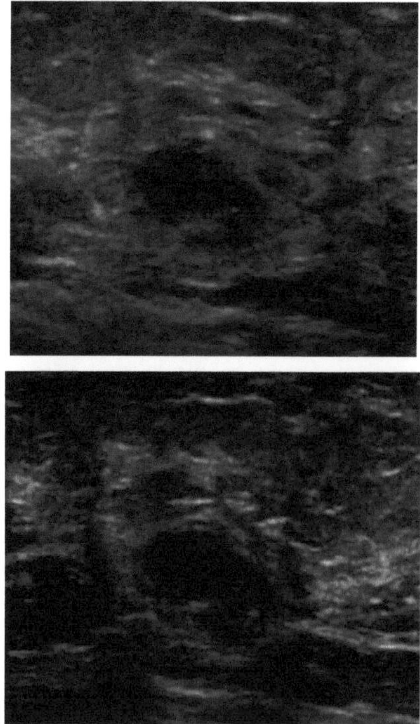

Fig. 14. Composite mode. (a) B-mode ultrasound. Hypoechoic mass, at
(b) Composite mode ultrasound. Hypoechoic, circumscribed mass. Histology:
Adenofibroma.

7. DOPPLER MODE

It is used to detect tumour angiogenesis. Malignant lesions are generally more vascularised than benign lesions, with an abnormal, irregular appearance of the vessels. Detection and analysis of the spectrum of these vessels requires a probe of at least 10 MHz and a rigorous ultrasound technique (adjustment of the focal length, reduction of the overall gain, adaptation of the size of the doppler box, filtering to the minimum 10 in order to analyse the low frequencies, no pressure on the breast to avoid obliteration of the small vessels) [32,33].

Energy Doppler has a better sensitivity to slow flows, but is more sensitive to artefacts [34]. Doppler can be used to analyse hypoechoic lesions which pose a "cystic or solid" problem. The presence of vascularisation in an echogenic lesion indicates that the lesion is tissue. On the other hand, the absence of vascularisation does not rule out the presence of a tissue portion [23] (fig. 15).

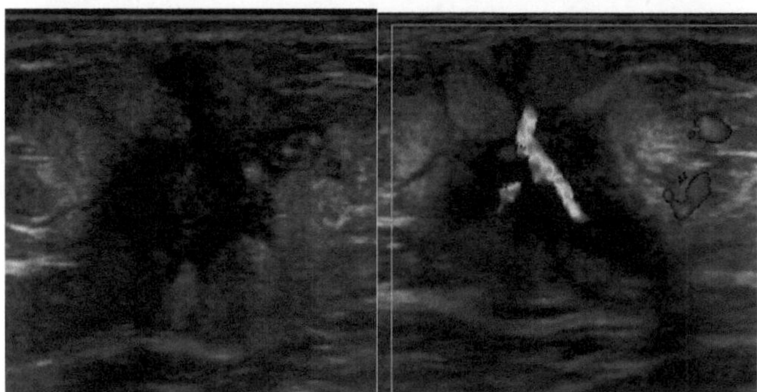

Fig. 15. Doppler mode (a) B-mode ultrasound. Contours spiculated, (b) Ultrasound mode The intralesional vascularisation.

8. ELASTOGRAPHY

Elastography is a non-invasive technique used in conjunction with ultrasound to qualitatively, semi-quantitatively or quantitatively assess the deformability of lesions subjected to stress [35, 36]. The image obtained is then translated into an elastogram. This technique was developed to improve the specificity of B-mode breast ultrasound by adding compressibility and lesion "hardness" to the criteria of echostructure and lesion morphology (fig. 16). Breast elastography uses two distinct modes: free-hand elastography and shear-wave elastography.

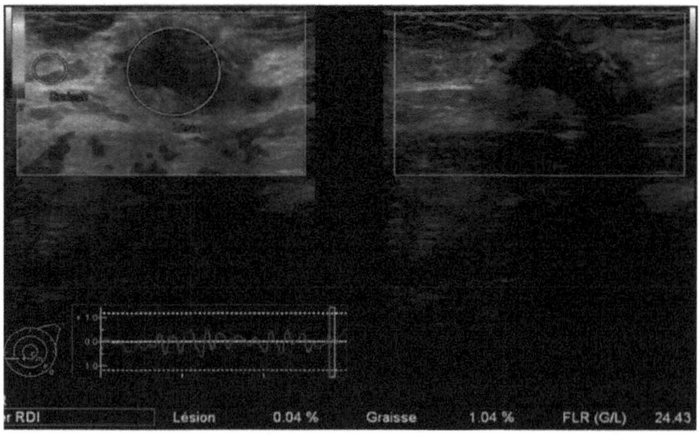

Fig. 16. elastography. Elastography. Calculation of the elasticity ratio in standard deviation.

MOLECULAR CLASSIFICATION IMAGING

1. LUMINAL TYPE A CANCER

On mammography, the stromal reaction developed around the tumour gives it a typical presentation in the form of a hyperdense, irregular mass, often spiculated in 37% of cases or with indistinct contours in 29% of cases [37, 38]. These cancers are particularly visible on tomosynthesis, especially as they are small (figs. 17, 18, 19). On ultrasound, their shape is usually irregular, with spiculated contours, a perilesional hyperechoic halo and posterior attenuation [37]. The posterior ultrasound attenuation is due to the fact that this is the molecular subtype with the most connective tissue compared with the other molecular subtypes [39] (figs. 17, 18, 19).The results of some elastography studies are divergent [40-55]. Jin Y et al [42] found that the highest elasticity ratio values were in luminal subtype A. According to Jin, tumour hardness correlates with desmoplastic reaction, which is important in luminal subtype A. However, Chang et al [43] showed that tumours with a mean low elasticity < 50 kPa were luminal subtypes (figs. 17, 18, 19).

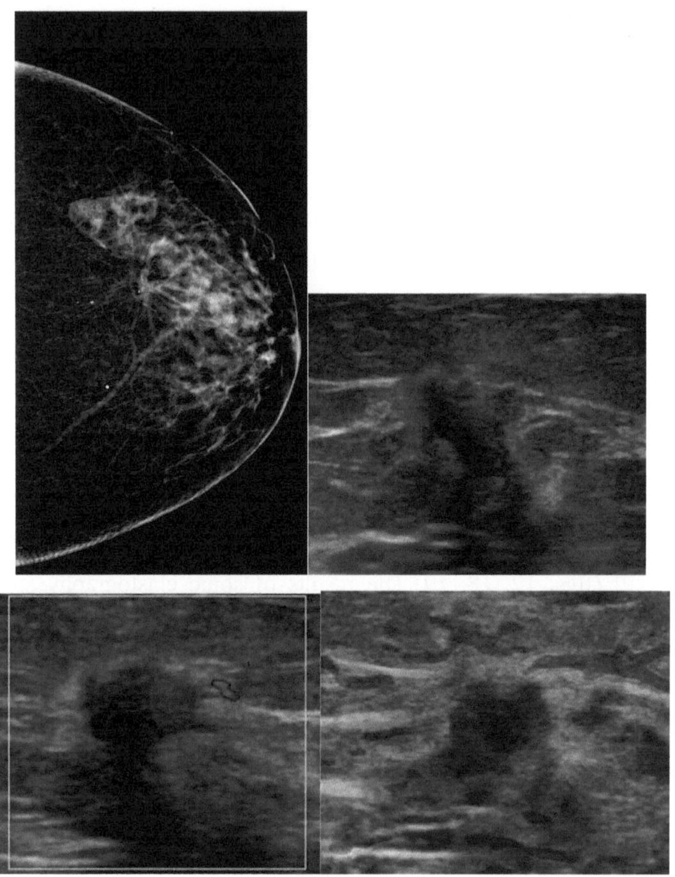

Fig. 17. luminal cancer A. Woman aged 54. (a) Mammogram. Hyperdense mass with spiculated contours (arrow). (b) B-mode ultrasound. Irregular, hypoechoic mass with spiculated contours, attenuating, surrounded by a peripheral echogenic halo (arrow) (c) Colour Doppler. Poorly vascularised mass. (d) Elastography. Hard mass, Itoh elasticity score 5. Histology: Invasive carcinoma NST grade I, RH +, HER2-, Ki 67 :13 %.

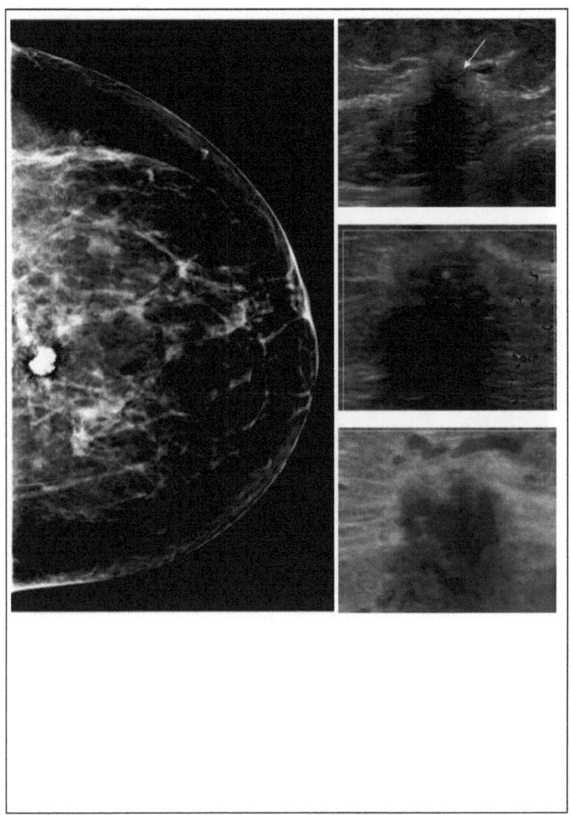

Fig. 18. luminal cancer A. Woman aged 58. (a) Mammogram. Hyperdense mass with spiculated contours (arrow). (b) B-mode ultrasound. Irregular, hypoechoic mass with spiculated contours, attenuating, surrounded by a peripheral echogenic halo (arrow). (c) Colour Doppler. Poorly vascularised mass.(d) Elastography. Hard mass with Itoh elasticity score 5. Histology: Invasive carcinoma NST grade I, RH +, HER2-, Ki 67: 5%.

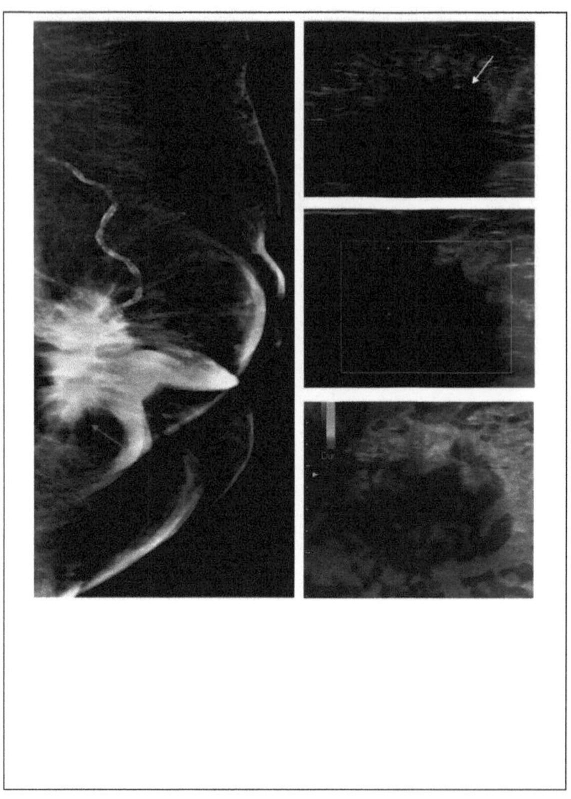

Fig. 19. luminal A cancer. Woman aged 77. (a) Mammogram. Hyperdense mass with spiculated contours (arrow) responsible for skin retraction. (b) B-mode ultrasound. Irregular, hypoechoic mass with spiculated contours, attenuating, surrounded by a peripheral echogenic halo (arrow). (c) Colour Doppler. Poorly vascularised mass. (d) Elastography. Hard mass with Itoh elasticity score 5. Histology: Invasive carcinoma NST grade II, RH +, HER2-, Ki 67: 14%.

2. LUMINAL TYPE B CANCER

These cancers do not have a typical presentation on imaging, but are very similar to luminal subtype A (figs. 20, 21, 22, 23, 24, 25, 26, 27). On mammography, this molecular type is more often found to have an irregular shape and indistinct contours [38]. On the other hand, the luminal B subtype with positive HR and positive HER2 may be spiculated in 27% of cases. However, it is architectural distortion that is most often associated [38].

On ultrasound, some studies have shown that there is no significant difference in radiological characteristics between the two luminal subtypes [52]. However, others have significantly observed an irregular shape in 88% of cases and posterior attenuation in 85% of cases [56]. The hyperechoic halo may be found in luminal B cancers but is less marked than in luminal A cancers [57].

On colour Doppler, the mass is often hypervascularised [58].

On elastography, some studies have shown that luminal tumours are less hard than other molecular types [41].

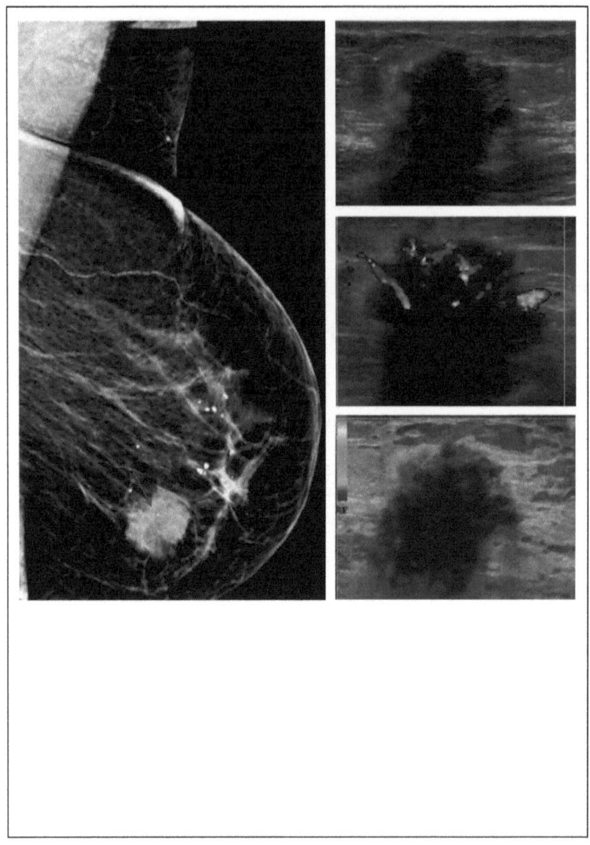

Fig. 20. luminal B cancer. Woman aged 48 (a) Mammogram. Irregularly shaped and contoured, hyperdense mass. (b) B-mode ultrasound. Irregularly shaped mass with indistinct contours, hypoechoic, heterogeneous, attenuating, surrounded by a discrete peripheral echogenic halo. (c) Colour Doppler. Hypervascularised mass. (d) Elastography. Hard mass, elasticity score 5. Histology: Invasive carcinoma NST grade II, RH +, HER2-, Ki 67: 30%.

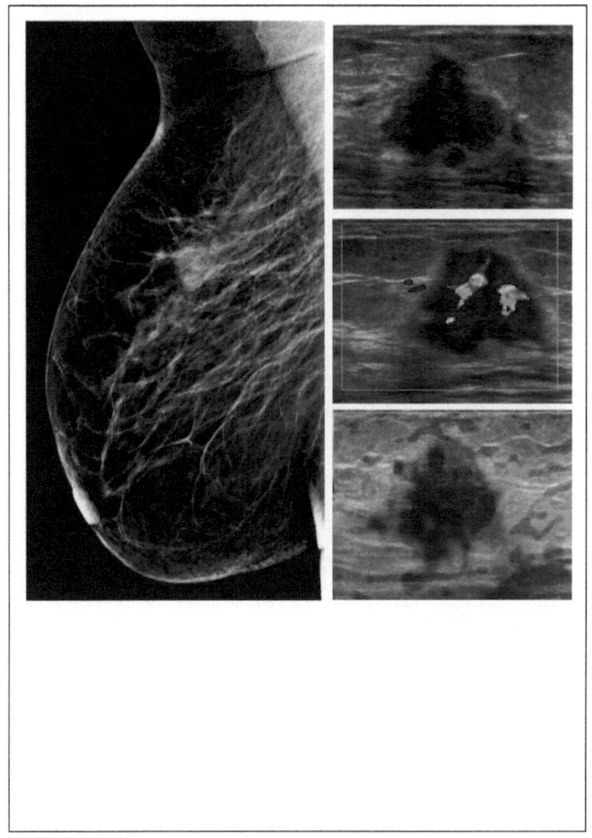

Fig. 21. luminal cancer B. 52-year-old woman(a) Mammogram. Mass of irregular shape and contours, hyperdense. (b) B-mode ultrasound. Irregularly shaped mass with irregular contours, hypoechoic, heterogeneous, discreetly attenuating, surrounded by a discrete peripheral echogenic halo. (c) Colour Doppler. Hypervascularised mass. (d) Elastography. Hard mass, elasticity score 5. Histology: Invasive carcinoma NST grade I, RH +, HER2-. Ki 67: 15%.

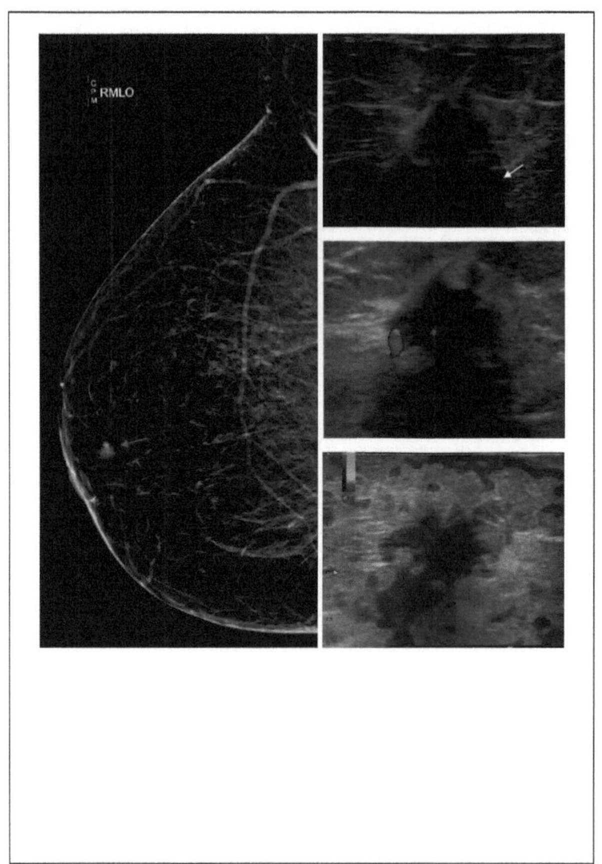

Fig. 22. luminal B cancer. Woman aged 48 (a) Mammogram. Mass of irregular shape and contours, isodense to glandular tissue. (b) B-mode ultrasound. Irregularly shaped mass with fine interface and posterior attenuation (arrow). (c) Colour Doppler. Peripheral vascularisation (d) Elastography. Hard mass. Histology: Invasive lobular carcinoma grade II, RH +, HER2-, Ki 67: 30%.

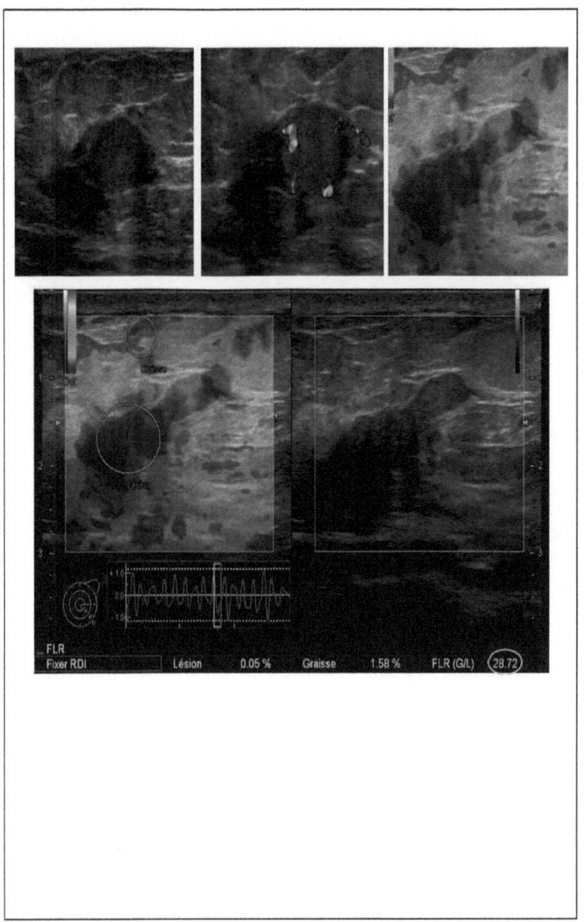

Fig. 23. luminal B cancer. Woman aged 47. (a) B-mode ultrasound. The mass is irregular in shape, with irregular contours, hypoechoic, homogeneous and with a thin interface, with no posterior acoustic effect. (b) Colour Doppler. Central and peripheral vascularisation (c+d) Elastography. Hard mass, elasticity score 5, high elasticity ratio. Histology: Invasive micro-papillary carcinoma grade II, RH +, HER2-, Ki 67: 50%.

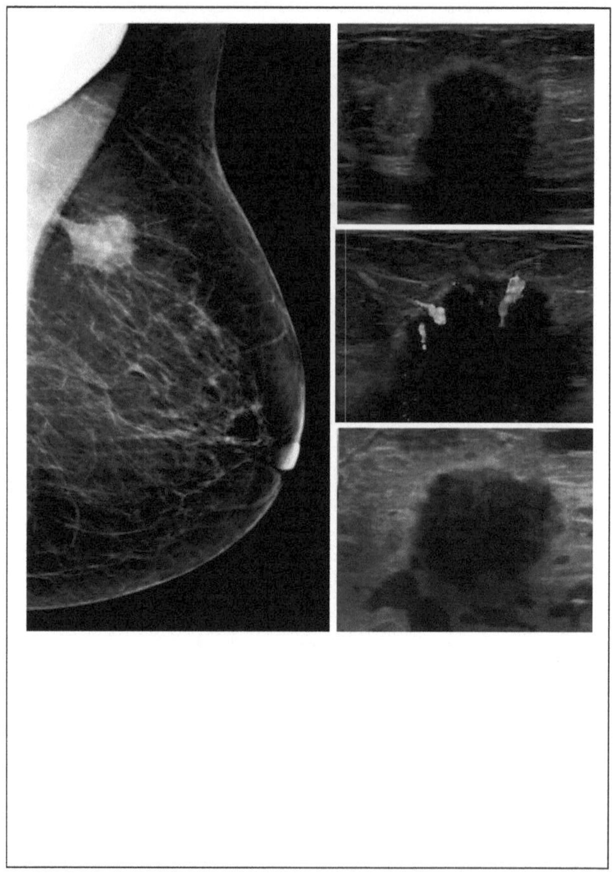

Fig. 24. luminal cancer B. Woman aged 67(a) Mammogram. Mass of irregular shape and contours, hyperdense. (b) B-mode ultrasound. Irregularly shaped mass with indistinct contours, hypoechoic, heterogeneous, attenuating, surrounded by a discrete peripheral echogenic halo. (c) Colour Doppler. Hypervascularised mass. (d) Elastography. Hard mass, elasticity score 5. Histology: Invasive carcinoma NST grade I, RH +, HER2-, Ki 67: 20%.

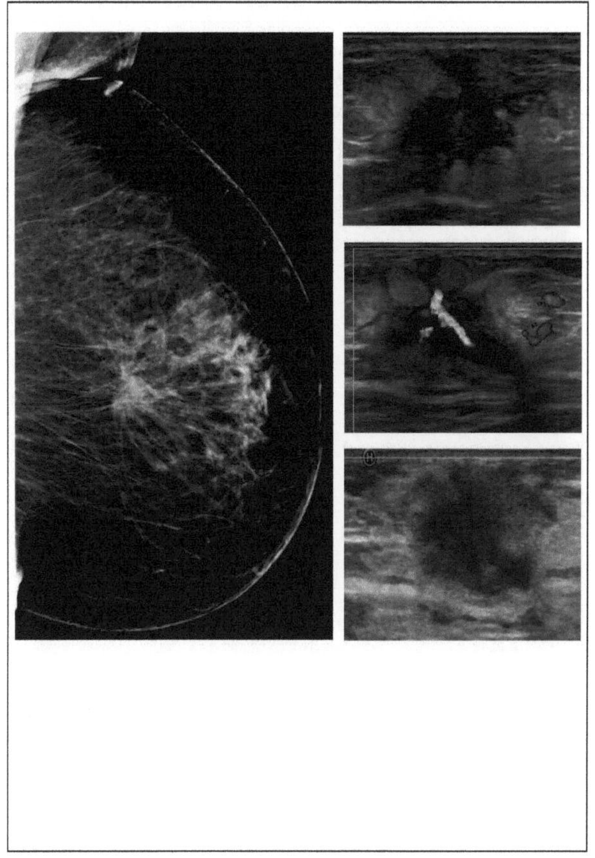

Fig. 25. luminal B cancer. Woman aged 52 (a) Mammogram. Irregularly shaped mass at the union of the quadrants, with spiculated contours, hyperdense (arrow). (b) B-mode ultrasound. Irregularly shaped mass with spiculated contours, hypoechoic, surrounded by a peripheral echogenic halo. (c) Colour Doppler. Hypervascularised mass. (d+e) Elastography. Hard lesion, score 5. Histology: Invasive carcinoma of NST grade II, RH +, HER2-, Ki 67: 20%.

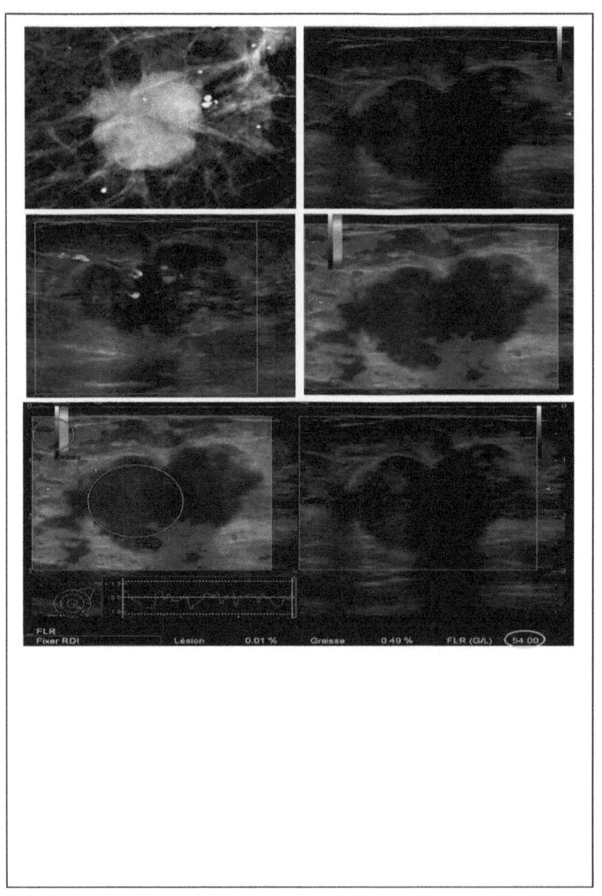

Fig. 26. B+HER2 luminal cancer. Woman aged 70 (a) Mammogram. Irregularly shaped and contoured mass, hyperdense. (b) B-mode ultrasound. Irregularly shaped mass with indistinct contours, hypoechoic, heterogeneous, attenuating, with abrupt interface. (c) Colour Doppler. Hypervascularised mass. (d+e) Elastography. Hard mass, elasticity score 5, very high elasticity ratio 54. Histology: Invasive carcinoma of NST grade II, RE +, RP -, HER2+, Ki 67: 40%.

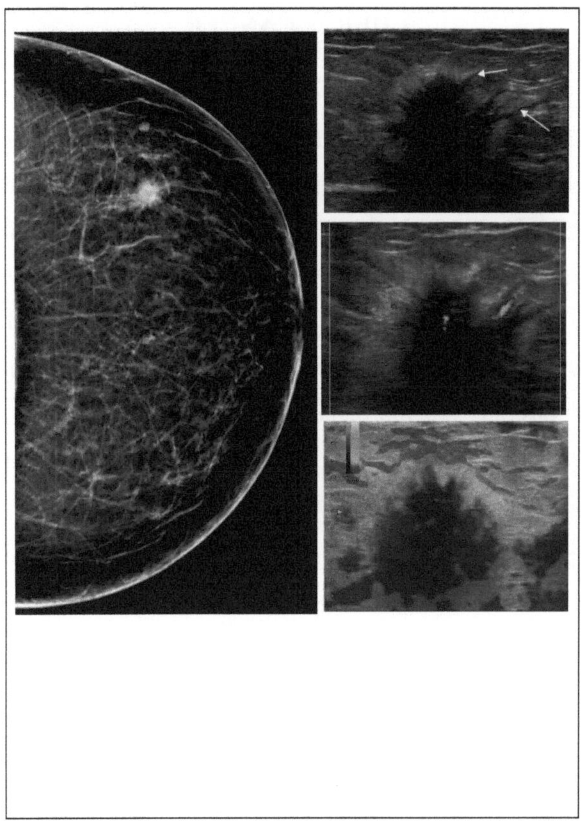

Fig. 27. Luminal cancer B+HER2. Woman aged 45 (a) Mammogram. Hyperdense, irregularly shaped mass with spiculated contours (arrow). (b) Ultrasound mode B. Irregular, hypoechoic mass with spiculated contours (arrows) with posterior attenuation, surrounded by a peripheral echogenic halo. (c) Colour Doppler. Vascularised mass. (d) Elastography. Mass with Itoh elasticity score 5. Histology: Invasive carcinoma NST grade II, RH +, HER2 +, Ki 67: 25%.

3. HER 2+ CANCER

On mammography, it is most frequently seen as an isodense mass with indistinct or sometimes circumscribed contours [37, 59]. HER2+ disease is often associated with ductal carcinoma in situ. In fact, the presence of suspicious microcalcifications on mammography is significantly associated with HER2 + status, so that the presence of microcalcifications is predictive of HER2 status when the HER2 score is equivocal 2+ on microbiopsy [60]. These microcalcifications are polymorphous, located in the mass or segmentally distributed [37] (fig. 28). On ultrasound, a rather irregular mass is seen, with indistinct contours and the interface between the tumour and the healthy parenchyma is often abrupt, angular, with no hyperechoic halo [37]. Posterior enhancement is often associated [52, 61]. These lesions are hypervascularised on colour Doppler [52, 61]. HER2+ status is closely linked to tumour angiogenesis, which may be due to increased expression of endothelial growth factor. Consequently, HER2+ cancers are often hypervascularised on colour Doppler (figs. 29, 30). Using elastography, many objective studies showed that the mean hardness of HER2 tumours was higher than that of luminal tumours [41, 43, 62] (fig. 31).

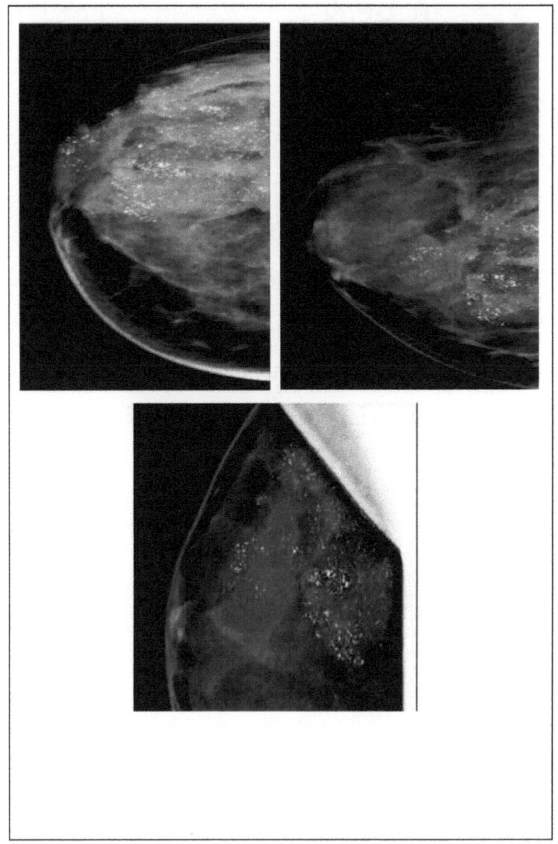

Fig. 28. HER2+ cancer. Woman aged 40. Mammography: (a) Front view (b) Oblique view (c) Enlargement. Extensive microcalcifications in the inferolateral quadrant, polymorphous and vermicular. Histology: Invasive carcinoma NST grade II, RH -, HER2 +.

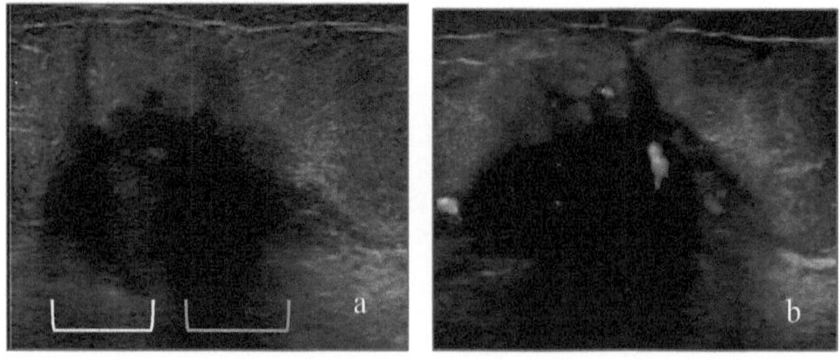

Fig. 29. HER2+ cancer. Woman aged 52. (a) B-mode ultrasound. (b) Colour Doppler. Irregularly shaped mass with angular contours, showing a mixed acoustic effect with posterior enhancement and attenuation (asterisk). Histology: Invasive carcinoma NST grade II, RH -, HER2 +, Ki67: 35%.

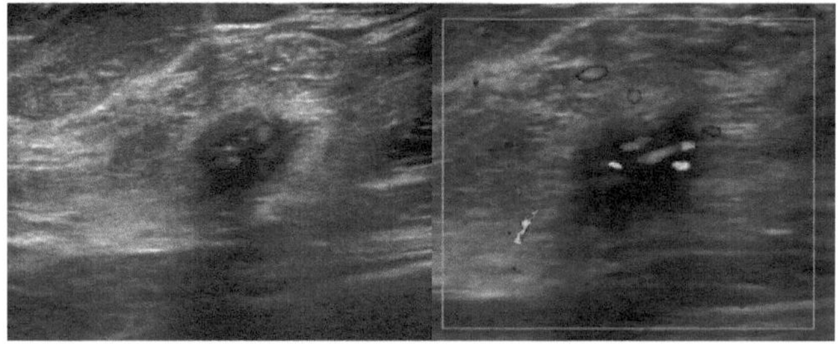

Fig. 30. HER2+ cancer. Woman aged 52 (a) B-mode ultrasound. (b) Doppler colour. Mass irregular, with contours angular, with calcifications (arrows), mixed posterior acoustic (enhancement +attenuation) and hypervascular at Doppler Histology :
Invasive carcinoma NST grade II, RH -, HER2 +, Ki67: 35%.

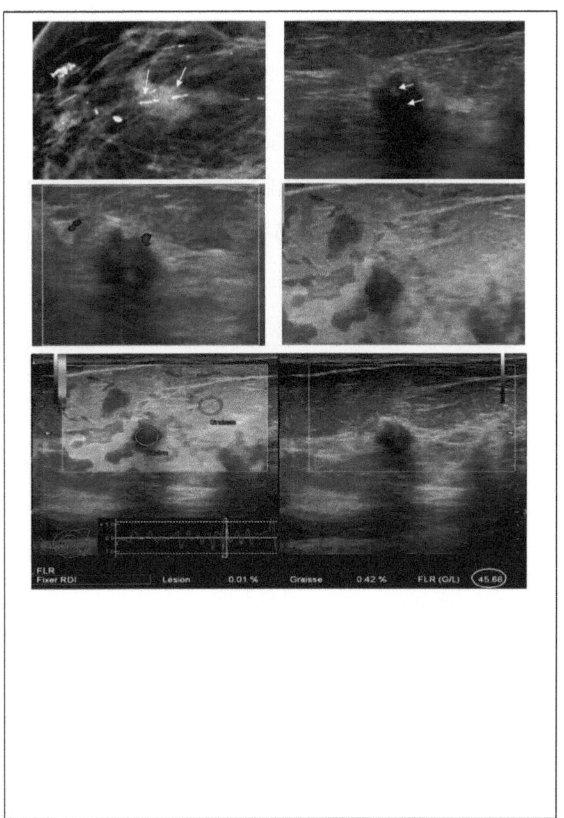

Fig. 31. HER2+ cancer. Woman aged 56 (a) Mammogram. Hyperdense, irregularly shaped mass with indistinct contours and calcifications within the mass (arrows). (b) B-mode ultrasound. Irregular mass with indistinct contours, hypoechoic, heterogeneous due to the presence of calcifications within it (arrows), with an abrupt interface and posterior attenuation. (c) Colour Doppler. Mass with peripheral vascularisation. (d+e) Elastography. Mass with an elasticity score of 5 and a high elasticity ratio of 45.66. Histology: Invasive carcinoma NST grade II, RH -, HER2 +, Ki 67: 30%.

4. TRIPLE-NEGATIVE CANCER

On mammography, the mass is the most common presentation, round or oval in 60-70% of cases, with well circumscribed or microlobulated contours in 24-43% of cases [37, 63]. There is little or no perilesional stromal reaction because of its rapid and aggressive course [52]. In fact, this tumour subtype does not go through a precancerous stage [37]. They are less often associated with ductal carcinoma in situ and are less likely to find microcalcifications on mammography at diagnosis [52, 61, 64, 65]. Focal asymmetry is more frequently found in triple-negative cancers than in luminal A and B subtypes [61]. The rate of normal mammograms in triple-negative cancers varies from 0 to 18%, probably due to the high breast density, which may mask the lesions, or to their rapid growth, which does not lead to architectural distortion [61, 66] (figs. 32, 33).On ultrasound, triple-negative cancers are very hypoechoic masses, found in 48% of cases, or heterogeneous masses with areas of necrosis, particularly when the long axis of the lesion exceeds 30 mm [61, 66]. These lesions often have smooth contours [57]. Posterior enhancement is found in 35.5% to 49% of cases [37, 61, 63]. Wu et al. found that triple-negative cancers were poorly vascularised on colour Doppler, and speculated that this was related to the central necrosis present [52, 60]. Kojima and Tsunoda showed that a colour Doppler signal was found in 90% of triple-negative tumours, but that it was most often a few vascular spots or pedicles [66]. These cancers often have pseudo-benign presentations, which explains why they are diagnosed at an advanced stage [64, 67] (figs. 32, 33, 34, 35). With regard to elastography, some studies in the literature have shown different results. Chang et al [43] evaluated 377 patients with invasive breast cancer and their mean elasticity values. They found that the elasticity values of triple-negative tumours were higher than those of luminal subtypes A and B (p < 0.0001). In the Youk et al study [62], on a series of 166 invasive breast cancers in 152 patients, the authors also showed that invasive HER2 and triple-negative cancers were harder than luminal subtype cancers (mean elasticity of triple-negative tumours 163.1 ± 47.6 kPa vs luminal A 135.2 ± 48.4 kPa, p = 0.009). In the Evans et al. series, triple-negative tumours had higher elasticity values of 169.1 ± 48.5 kPa than luminal tumours (136.9 ± 57.2 kPa). According to Evans, tissue hardness appears to be statistically significantly correlated with tumour aggressiveness [41]. Furthermore, Ganau et al [47] reported that aggressive phenotypes (triple-negative and HER2 status) appear to have moderately lower elasticity than less aggressive phenotypes (luminal A and luminal B), but without significant difference. Denis et al [47] reported that the triple-negative subtype had the lowest elasticity values (44.6 kPa triple-negative vs 108 kPa luminal A). Similarly, Jin Y et al [42] found that the lowest elasticity ratio values were in triple-negative tumours, respectively 75,58. The highest values were for luminal A and B subtypes, 90.69 and 81.86 respectively (p < 0.0001).

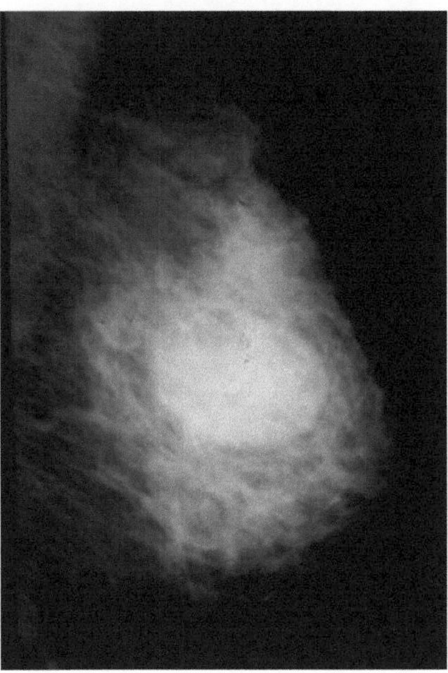

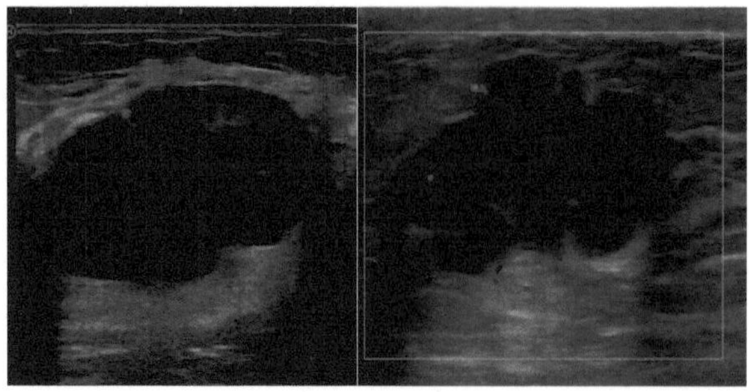

Fig. 32. triple-negative cancer. Woman aged 56 (a) Mammogram. Hyperdense mass, roughly oval in shape, with circumscribed contours (arrow). (b) B-mode ultrasound. An oval mass with microlobulated contours, highly hypoechoic, with an abrupt interface and posterior enhancement (arrow). (c) Colour Doppler. Poorly vascularised mass. Histology: Carcinoma infiltrating NST grade III, RH -, HER2 -.

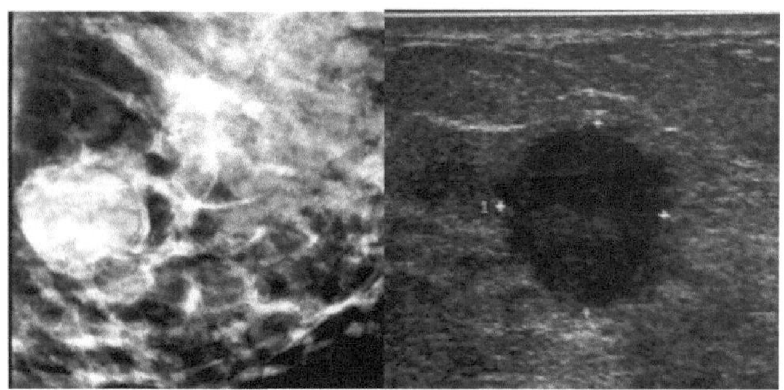

Fig. 33. triple-negative cancer. Woman aged 43 (a) Mammogram. Round, circumscribed, hyperdense mass (arrow). (b) Ultrasound mode B. Round mass with microlobulated contours, strongly hypoechoic, with abrupt interface and posterior enhancement (arrow). Histology: Invasive carcinoma NST grade III, RH -, HER2 -.

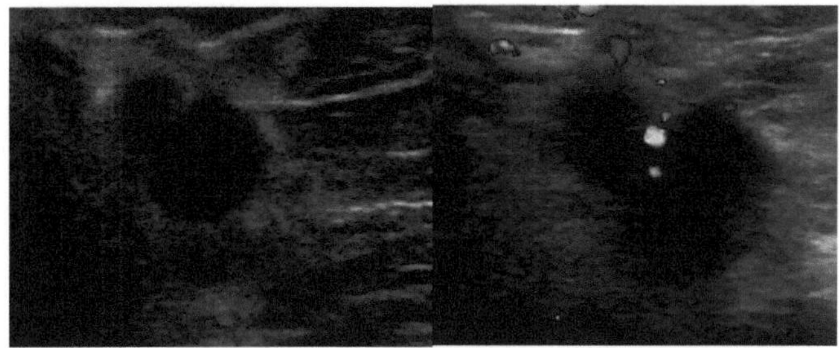

Fig. 34. triple-negative cancer. Woman aged 57. (a) B-mode ultrasound. A circumscribed mass with microlobulated contours, highly hypoechoic, with an abrupt interface and posterior enhancement (arrow). (b) Colour Doppler. Poorly vascularised mass. Histology: Invasive carcinoma NST grade II, RH -,HER2 -.

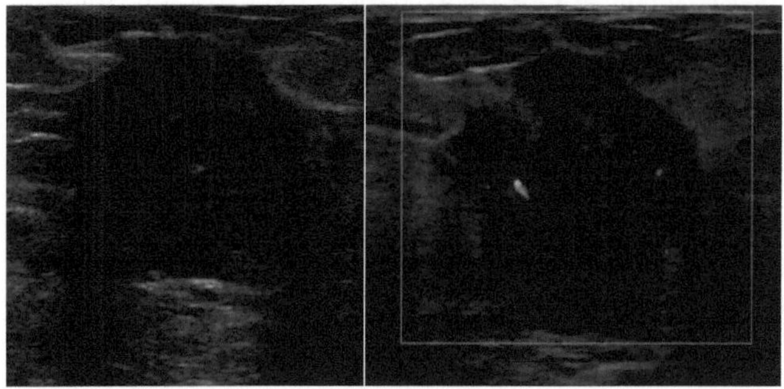

Fig. 35. Triple-negative cancer. Woman aged 78. (a) B-mode ultrasound. A circumscribed mass with microlobulated contours, highly hypoechoic, with an abrupt interface and posterior enhancement (arrow). (b) Colour Doppler. Poorly vascularised mass. Histology: Invasive carcinoma NST grade II, RH -,

HER2 -.

REFERENCES

1. Putti TC, El-Rehim DM, Rakha EA, Paish CE, Lee AH, Pinder SE, Ellis IO. Estrogen receptor-negative breast carcinomas: a review of morphology and immunophenotypical analysis. Mod Pathol. 2005 Jan;18(1):26-35.

2. Carey LA, Dees EC, Sawyer L, Gatti L, Moore DT, Collichio F, Ollila DW, Sartor CI, Graham ML, Perou CM. The triple negative paradox: primary tumor chemosensitivity of breast cancer subtypes. Clin Cancer Res. 2007 Apr 15;13(8):2329-34.

3. Lakhani SR, Ellis IO, Schnitt SJ, Tan PH, van de Vijver MJ (Eds.): WHO Classification of Tumours of the Breast. IARC: Lyon 2012.

4. Elston CW, Ellis IO. Pathological prognostic factors in breast cancer. I. The value of histological grade in breast cancer: experience from a large study with long- termfollow-up. Histopathology 1991;19:403-10.

5. Putti TC, El-Rehim DM, Rakha EA, et al. Estrogen receptor-negative breast carcinomas: a review of morphology and immunophenotypical analysis. Mod Pathol 2005;18:26-35.

6. Parl FF, Schmidt BP, Dupont WD, Wagner RK. Prognostic significance of estrogen receptor status in breast cancer in relation to tumor stage, axillary node metastasis, and histopathologic grading. Cancer 1984;54: 2237-2242.

7. Carey LA, Dees EC, Sawyer L, et al. The triple negative paradox: primary tumor chemosensitivity of breast cancer subtypes. Clin Cancer Res 2007;13:2329-2334.

8. Prat, A., Ellis, M. J., and Perou, C. M. Practical implications of gene-expression- based assays for breast oncologists. Nature reviews Clinical oncology, 2012: 9(1), 48-57.

9. Goldhirsch A, Winer EP, Coates AS, Gelber RD, Piccart-Gebhart M,

Th'äö¬ʃrlimann B, Senn HJ; Panel members. Personalizing the treatment of women with early breast cancer: highlights of the St Gallen International Expert Consensus on the Primary Therapy of Early Breast Cancer 2013. Ann Oncol. 2013 Sep;24(9):2206-23. doi: 10.1093/annonc/mdt303. Epub 2013.

10. Billar JA, Dueck AC, Stucky CC, Gray RJ, Wasif N, Nothfelts D. Triple-negative breast cancers: unique clinical presentations and outcomes. Ann Surg Oncol 2010;17:384-90.

11. Whitman GJ, Albarracin CT, Gonzalez-Angulo AM. Triple negative breast cancer: what the radiologist needs to know. Semin Roentgenol 2011;46(1):26-39.

12. Baur A, Bahrs SD, Speck S, Wietek BM, Kremer B, Vogel U, et al. Breast MRI of pure ductal carcinoma in situ: sensitivity of diagnosis and influence of lesion characteristics. Eur J Radiol 2013;82:1731-7.

13. Hammersleya JA, Partridgeb SC, Blitzera GC, Deitcha S, Rahbarb H. Management of high-risk breast lesions found on mammogram or ultrasound: the value of contrast-enhanced MRI to exclude malignancy. Clinical Imaging 49; 2018; 174-180. https://doi.org/10.1016/j.clinimag.2018.03.011

14. Andolina VF, Lill√© SL, Willison KM, Mammographic Imaging. A practical guide. 2 nd ed. Lippincott Williams and Wilkins; 2001.

15. Austin C. R and Short R. V. Hormonal Control of Reproduction. 2nd edition of Reproduction in Mammals, Vol.3. Cambridge: Cambridge University Press. 1984.

16. Faulconer LS, Parham CA, Connor DM, Kuzmiak C, et al. Effect of breast compression on lesion characteristic visibility with diffraction-enhanced imaging. Acad Radiol 2010; 17 (4) : 433-40. Epub 2009 Dec 29.

17. Kinzelin S. Positioning, the √©tape cl√© of the mammography examination. Imagerie du sein Elsevier Masson, 2012; 2: 19-27.

18. Mancuso S, Ottolenghi G. The oblique projection in the radiologic Study of the breast. Minerva Ginecol 1989; 41 (7): 325-8.

19. Konguth PJ, Rimer BK, Conaway MR, et al. Impact of patient-controlled compression on the mammography experience. Radiology 1993; 186 (1): 99-102.

20. Muntz EP, Logan WW, Focal spot size. And scatter supression in magnification mammography. AJR Am J Roentgenol 1979; 133 (3): 453-9.

21. Corsetti V, Houssami N, Ferrari A, Ghirardi M, Bellarosa S, Angelini O, et al. Breast screening with ultrasound in women with mammography-negative dense breasts: evidence on incremental cancer detection and false positives, and associated cost. Eur J Cancer. 2008 Mar;44(4):539-44.

22. Athanasiou A, Tardivon A, Ollivier L, Thibault F, El Khoury C, Neuenschwander S. How to optimize breast ultrasound. Eur J Radiol. 2009 Jan;69(1):6-13.

23. Weinstein SP, Conant EF, Sehgal C. Technical advances in breast ultrasound imaging. Semin Ultrasound CT MR. 2006 Aug;27(4):273-83.

24. Sehgal CM, Weinstein SP, Arger PH, Conant EF. A review of breast ultrasound. J Mammary Gland Biol Neoplasia. 2006 Apr;11(2):113-23.

25. Amersham Health. Encyclopaedia of Medical Imaging. http://eu.aershamhealth/com/medcyclopaedia/

26. Clevert DA, Jung EM, Jungius KP, Ertan K, Kubale R. Value of tissue harmonic imaging (THI) and contrast harmonic imaging (CHI) in detection and characterisation of breast tumours. Eur Radiol 2007 ; 17 : 1-10.

27. Rosen EL, Soo MS. Tissue harmonic imaging sonography of breast lesions: improved margin analysis, conspicuity, and image quality compared to conventional ultrasound. Clin Imaging. 2001 Nov-Dec;25(6):379-84.

28. Athanasiou A, Balleyguier C. New techniques in breast ultrasound. Imagerie de la Femme. 2007;17(4):247-54.

29. Huber S, Wagner M, Medl M, Czembirek H. Real-time spatial compound imaging in breast ultrasound. Ultrasound Med Biol 2002; 28: 155-63.

30. Cha JH, Moon WK, Cho N, Chung SY, Park SH, Park JM, et al. Differentiation of benign from malignant solid breast masses: conventional US versus compound imaging. Radiology 2005;237:841-6.

31. Balu-Maestro C. Bases de l'√©chographie mammaire. Imager ie du sein. Paris: Elsevier-Masson; 2012. p. 101-17.

32. Dickinson RJ, Hill CR. Measurement of soft tissue motion using correlation between A-scans.Ultrasound Med Biol 1982;8(3):263-71.

33. Krouskop TA, Dougherty DR, Vinson FS. A pulsed Doppler ultrasonic system for making noninvasive measurements of the mechanical properties of soft tissue. J Rehabil Res Dev 1987;24(2):1-8.

34. Ophir J, Cépedes I, Ponnekanti H, Yazdi Y, Li X. Elastography: a quantitative method for imaging the elasticity of biological tissues. Ultrason Imaging 1991;13(2):111-34.

35. Youk JH, Gweon HM, Son EJ. Shear-wave elastography in breast ultrasonography: the state of the art. Ultrasonography. 2017 Oct;36(4):300-309. doi: 10.14366/usg.17024.

36. Tristant H, Benmussa M, Bokobsa J, Elbaz P. Variation of the normal breast: mammographic and ultrasonographic aspects. Encycl Méd Chir 1994; 810-G-15.

37. Boisserie-Lacroix M, Hurtevent-Labrot G, Ferron S, Lippa N, Bonnefoi H, Mac Grogan G. Correlation between imaging and molecular classification of breast cancers. Diagn Interv Imaging 2013;94(11):1069-80.

38. Au FW-F, Ghai S, Lu F-I, Moshonov H, Crystal P. Histological grade and

immunohistochemical biomarkers of breast cancer: correlation to ultrasound features: breast cancer grade and biomarkers correlated to ultrasound features. J Ultrasound Med 2017;36(9):1883-94.

39. Kobayashi T. Diagnostic ultrasound in breast cancer: analysis of retrotumorous echo patterns correlated with sonic attenuation by cancerous connective tissue. J Clin Ultrasound 1979;7(6):471-9.

40. Grajo JR, Barr RG. Strain elastography for prediction of breast cancer tumor grades. J Ultrasound Med. 2014 Jan;33(1):129-34.

41. Evans A, Whelehan P, Thomson K, McLean D, Brauer K, Purdie C, et al. Invasive breast cancer: relationship between shear-wave elastographic findings and histologic prognostic factors. Radiology. 2012;263(3):673-7.

42. Jin Y, Fenghua L, Jing D, Yifen G. Strain elastography features in invasive breast cancer: relationship between stiffness and pathological factors. Int J Clin Exp Med 2017;10(9):13290-13297.

43. Chang JM, Park IA, Lee SH, Kim WH, Bae MS, Koo HR, et al. Stiffness of tumors measured by shear-wave elastography correlated with subtypes of breast cancer. Eur Radiol 2013;23(9):2450-8.

44. Durhan G, ũztekin PS, únverdi H et al. Do Histopathological Features and Microcalcification Affect the Elasticity of Breast Cancer? J Ultrasound Med. 2017 Jun;36(6):1101-1108.

45. Ganau S, Andreu FJ, Escribano F, et al. Shear-wave elastography and immunohistochemical profiles in invasive breast cancer: evaluation of maximum and mean elasticity values. Eur J Radiol 2015; 84:617-622.

46. Hayashi M, Yamamoto Y et al. Associations Between Elastography Findings and Clinicopathological Factors in Breast Cancer. Medicine. 2015, 94(50): e2290.

47. Denis M, Gregory A, Bayat M, Fazzio RT, Whaley DH, Ghosh K, Shah S,

Fatemi M and Alizad A. Correlating Tumor Stiffness with Immuno histochemical Subtypes of Breast Cancers: prognostic value of Comb-Push ultrasound shear elastography for differentiating luminal subtypes. PLoS One 2016; 11: e0165003.

48. Romero Q, Bendahl, PO, Fernö M, Grabau D and Borgquist S. A novel model for Ki67 assessment in breast cancer. Diagn. Pathol. 9, 118 (2014).

49. Galant C, Berlière M, Leconte I, Marbaix E. Novelty in histopronostic factors in breast cancer. Imagerie de la Femme (2010) 20, 9-17.

50. Liu Y, Huang Y, Han J, Wang J, et al. Association Between Shear Wave Elastography of Virtual Touch Tissue Imaging Quantification Parameters and the Ki-67 Proliferation Status in Luminal-Type Breast Cancer. J Ultrasound Med 2018; 00:00-00, 0278-4297.

51. Dominković MD, Ivanac G, Kelava T, Brklja_f_çi_f_á B et al. Elastographic features of triple negative breast cancers Eur Radiol (2016) 26:1090-1097. DOI 10.1007/s00330-015-3925-7.

52. Wua T, Lib J, Wanga D, Lenga X, ZhangaL et al. Identification of a correlation between the sonographic appearance and molecular subtype of invasive breast cancer: A review of 311 cases. Clinical Imaging 53 (2019) 179-185.

53. Wang D, Zhu K, Tian J, Li Z et al. Clinicopathological and Ultrasonic Features of Triple-Negative Breast Cancers: A Comparison with Hormone Receptor- Positive/Human Epidermal Growth Factor Receptor-2-Negative Breast Cancers. J Ultrasound Med Biol. 2018 May;44(5):1124-1132.

54. Li Z, Tian J, Wang X, Wang Y, Wang Z, Zhang L, Jing H, Wu T. Differences in multi-modal ultrasound imaging between triple negative and non-triple negative breast cancer. Ultrasound Med Biol 2016; 42:882-890

55. Sohn YM, Seo M. Breast lesions diagnosed by ultrasound-guided core needle biopsy: Can shearwave elastography predict histologic upgrade after surgery or vacuum assisted excision?". Clinical Imaging 49 (2018) 150-155.

56. Au-Yong IT, Evans AJ, Taneja S, Rakha EA, Green AR, Paish C, et al. Sonographic correlations with the new molecular classification of invasive cancer. Eur Radiol 2009;19: 2342-8.

57. Van Zelst JCM, Balkenhol M, Tan T, Rutten M, Imhof-Tas M, Bult P, et al. Sonographic phenotypes of molecular subtypes of invasive ductal cancer in automated 3-D breast ultrasound. Ultrasound Med Biol 2017;43(9):1820-8.

58. Zhang L, Li J, Xiao Y, Cui H, Du G, Wang Y, Li Z, Wu T, Li X, Tian J. Identifying ultrasound and clinical features of breast cancer molecular subtypes by ensemble decision. Sci Rep. 2015 Jun 5;5:11085.

59. Wu M, Zhong X, Peng Q, Xu M, Huang S, Yuan J, et al. Prediction of molecular subtypes of breast cancer using BI-RADS features based on a "white box" machine learning approach in a multimodal imaging setting. Eur J Radiol 2019;114:175- 84.

60. Shin HJ, Kim HH, Huh MO, Kim MJ, Yi A, Kim H, et al. Correlation between mammographic and sonographic findings and prognostic factors in patients with node-negative invasive breast cancer. Br J Radiol 2011;84(997):19-30.

61. Ko ES, Lee BH, Kim H-A, Noh W-C, Kim MS, Lee S-A. Triplenegative breast cancer: correlation between imaging and pathological findings. Eur Radiol 2010;20(5):1111-7.

62. Youk JH, Gweon HM, Son EJ, Kim JA, Jeong J. Shear-wave elastography of invasive breast cancer: correlation between quantitative mean elasticity value and immunohistochemical profile. Breast Cancer Res Treat 2013; 138:119-126.

63. Aho M, Irshad A, Ackerman SJ, Lewis M, Leddy R, Pope TL, et al. Correlation of sonographic features of invasive ductal mammary carcinoma with age, tumor grade, and hormone-receptor status. J Clin Ultrasound 2013;41(1):10-7.

64. Krizmanich-Conniff KM, Paramagul C, Patterson SK, Helvie MA, Roubidoux MA, Myles JD, et al. Triple receptor-negative breast cancer: imaging clinical characteristics. Am J Roentgenol 2012;199(2):458-64.

65. Yang W-T, Dryden M, Broglio K, Gilcrease M, Dawood S, Dempsey PJ, et al. Mammographic features of triple receptor-negative primary breast cancers in young premenopausal women. Breast Cancer Res Treat 2008;111(3):405-10.

66. Kojima Y, Tsunoda H. Mammography and ultrasound features of triple-negative breast cancer. Breast Cancer 2011;18(3):146-51.

67. Collett K. A basal epithelial phenotype is more frequent in interval breast cancers compared with screen detected tumors. Cancer Epidemiol Biomarkers Prev 2005;14(5):1108-12.

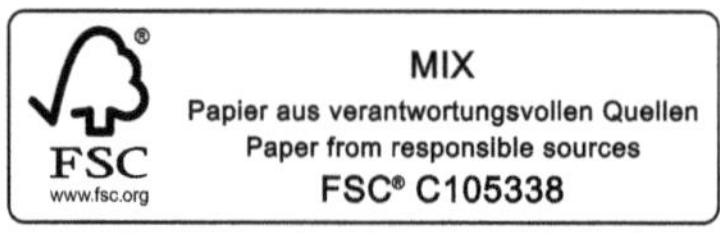

Printed by Books on Demand GmbH, Norderstedt / Germany